GreenPrint Diet Cookbook: Quick and Easy Plant-Based Diet Recipes to help you Lose weight and Feel Great.

by Laura Smith

Disclaimer:

PLEASE NOTE: This cookbook was not written, endorsed or approved by Marco Borges or Penguin Group (USA) LLC. The author of this cookbook is a firm believer in the Greenprint Diet and is passionate about sharing her unique and tasty recipes with the world.

The information provided in this book is designed to provide helpful information on the subjects discussed. The publisher and author are not responsible for any specific health or allergy needs that may require medical supervision and are not liable for any damages or negative consequences from any treatment, action, application or preparation, to any person reading or following the information in this book.

Download Your Free Gift Here>>

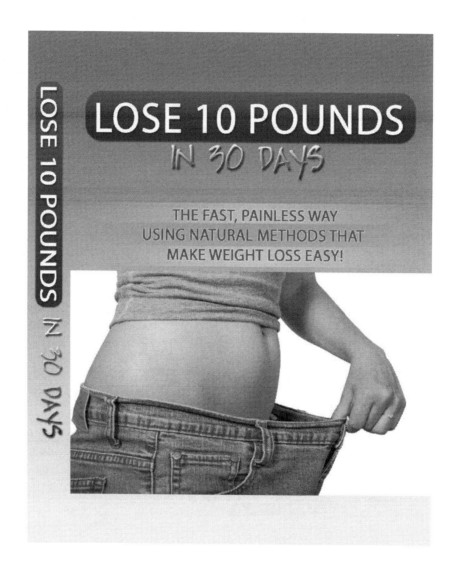

Discover how you Can Lose 10 Pounds in 30 Days or Less

with Over 100 Recipes you can Try Today!

Visit>> https://forms.aweber.com/form/23/167298623.htm

Contents

Introduction **8**

The Advantages of Going on the Plant-Based Diet **10**

Soaking methods & cooking recipes for Plant-Based staple foods **11**

Important Recipes **14**

Apple Sauce 14

Peanut Butter 15

Almond Milk 16

Breakfast **18**

Greenprint Breakfast Oat 18

Berry-Bana Smoothie Bag 19

Delicious Matcha Morning 20

Powerhouse Protein Shake 21

Mango Blaster Smoothie Bag 22

Peachy Mango Bowl 23

Main Dishes **24**

Vegetable Broth 25

Tortilla Wraps 27

Black Bean Soup 28

One Pan Ratatouille 30

Five- Grain Cereal with Apples, Bananas and Apricots 31

Pan Crisped Tofu with Greens and Peanut Dressing 32

Vegetable Tagine with Baked Tempe 33

Quinoa Tabbouleh 35

Potato Curry with Roti or Rice 36

Koshari 37

Seitan Stir fry with Black Bean Garlic Sauce 39

Barbecued Tempe Sandwiches with Peppers and Onion 40

Easy Vegetable Paella 41

Easy Mexican Freekeh Pilaf 42

Tempeh Rendang 43

Peanut Sauce Stir fry with Tempeh 44

Moroccan Flatbreads 45

Tofu Banh Mi 46

Pizzas and Pastas 46

Cilantro Basil Pesto Pasta 47

Coconut and Garlic White Pizza 48

Healthy Spinach Pine Nut Pizza 49

Tempeh- Pasta Casserole 50

Vegetable Arugula Whole Wheat Pizza 51

Soups and Salads 52

Easy Roasted Butternut Squash Soup 53

Moroccan Red Gazpacho 54

Apple Beet Soup 55

Red Lentil Carrot Soup 56

Asian Spring Vegetable Soup with Tofu 57

Antioxidant Cherry Fruit Salad 58

Watermelon and Heirloom Tomato Salad 59

Beluga Black Lentil Salad with Rice 60

Vegan Pasta Salad with Lime 61

Mango Bean Salsa 62

Appetizers and Snacks 63

Tofu Steaks with Red Pepper - Walnut Sauce 64

Portobello Fritte 65

South West Puff Pastry Bites 66

Vegetable and Garlic Stuffed Mushrooms 67

Vegan Spinach Balls 68

Beluga Black Lentil Burgers 69

Coconut Beet Patties 70

Tempeh Stuffed Butternut Squash 71

Sweet Potato Burgers 72

Vegan Egg Rolls 73

Avocado Hummus 75

Quick Roasted Garlic bread 76

Desserts **77**

    Banana-Oat Cups 78

    Raspberry Lemon Ice-Cream 79

    Mexikale Crisps 80

    Black Bean & Quinoa Burgers 81

    Peanut Butter Brownies 83

    Vegan Blueberry Lime Cheese Cake 84

    Vegan Chocolate Strawberry Cupcakes 86

    Vegan Mint Chocolate Mousse 88

    Vegan Peanut Butter Mousse Pie 88

    Apple Banana Muffins (with Streusel) 90

    Vegan Coconut Banana Cheesecake 91

    Vegan Kiwi Mango Cheesecake 92

    Nut Butter Cranberry Cookies 93

Conclusion **94**

Thank You **96**

Other Health And Fitness Bestselling Books ..... Error! Bookmark not defined.

Introduction

This diet is about the plant power, originated by the plant based Guru. In this greenprint plant based diet, he states that it's really important to understand that every time we eat we're either feeding disease or fueling health, right? It's really about elevating consciousness. It's not about labeling a diet, it's about saying, to ourselves, and acknowledging that, the more we lean towards plants, the greater the benefit.

The greenprint is exactly that. They've set 22 laws to help you, as guide rails to live your best life.

 ➢ You'll lose weight effortlessly.
 ➢ You'll transform your body.
 ➢ You're going to improve the planet.

So it's really about just eating more consciously, because every time we eat, we make a decision towards health.

In this Diet, the Number one rule is eat more, weigh less. The beauty about plant based diet is that, plant based foods have a high nutrient density but a very low calorie density, in that you are going to eat more and weigh less. However, plant based and vegan are pretty much the same thing, but a lot of people dreads vegan, while the plant based is quite accepted.

Plant Based Diet Contains Foods THAT ARE UNPROCESSED for example BEANS, LEGUMES, FRUITS, BEANS, LEGUMES, FRUITS, VEGETABLES, and these are SIMPLE FOODS THAT NOURISH YOU FROM THE INSIDE OUT. Not only is it easy to find, but it's actually less expensive to cook this away than to cook with meat products.

Nevertheless, the most important rule in this diet is to protect your heart. HEART DISEASE REMAINS THE NUMBER ONE KILLER, NOT JUST IN THE U.S. BUT AROUND the world. IT'S BECOME A $1 TRILLION PROBLEM, AND WE NEED TO PROTECT OUR HEARTS WITH THE FOOD THAT WE

EAT. Hence, PLANT-BASED DIET IS ONE OF THE BEST WAYS YOU CAN PROTECT YOUR HEART, because you are taking in all the nutrients that you need and Eliminating the cholesterol, and the saturated fats.

Now YOU CAN REVERSE DISEASE BY EATING HEALTHIER, because EVERY SINGLE DAY IS AN OPPORTUNITY TO LIVE THE LIFE YOU truly want to live.

The Advantages of Going on the Plant-Based Diet

One of greatest ideas behind the Greenprint Diet is "going Plant-Based". Dieters can enjoy considerable health benefits by adopting this lifestyle. Here are some of the advantages of adopting a plant-based diet:

Enough Protein: By mixing up protein sources with nuts, and beans, seeds, fruits, people on the plant based diet can enjoy the same vitamins and nutrients as meat eaters. Plant-based sources of protein provide the full spectrum of essential amino acids to ensure a healthy body.

It Helps Your Heart: According to a study in the American Journal of Clinical Nutrition, individuals on a plant-based diet have an average of 44% lower LDL cholesterol than those on a meat-based diet.

It Helps The Environment: One acre of land can produce just 165 pounds of beef or 20,000 pounds of potatoes. Come to think about this, going plant based will not only help you lose weight and get in shape, but will also help preserve the Environment.

You Don't Need Supplements: Many vegans take a supplement to ensure they're getting all of their recommended daily nutrients and vitamins. However, the greenprint Diet explains that it's not necessary, and that those who carefully follow a plant based diet will get all of the vitamins and nutrients they need.

In this Diet Recipe Book, We have prepared great tasting plant-based foods for your ultimate enjoyment. Eat more, while you lose weight and feel great.

Soaking methods & cooking recipes for Plant-Based staple foods

A few Plant-based ingredients come up time again in this Plant-Based recipe book and are always good to have on hand. These ingredients are ideal for adding texture, flavor, fiber and protein to your meals. Amongst them are beans, grains, nuts, seeds, oil, dried fruits and vegetables. Some of these (seeds, nuts and fruits) are also great to have as snacks.

Overnight soak

Leaving beans, lentils and legumes in a pot of water overnight (at least 8 hours) is the most effective way to soak. Use roughly 10 cups of water for every pound of dry beans (roughly 2 cups). Required soaking times are shown in the table below.

Soaking

Black Beans, lentils and split peas are rich in protein and fiber and are incorporated into many vegan recipes. However, they require soaking before cooking in order to be softened. This reduces the cooking time needed and helps digestion. Many of the 'anti-nutrients' found in beans are water-soluble, so they're removed during soaking. Anti-nutrients prevent nutrient absorption in the gastrointestinal tract. An alternative to soaking is sprouting.

These methods are explained in the tables below.

Hot soak

This is the quickest soaking method. Fill up a pot large enough to accommodate your beans or legumes with water. Add about 10 cups for each pound (roughly 2 cups) of dry beans, or make sure beans/legumes are covered with an excess of about 1 inch of water. Bring the water to a boil and allow it to simmer for about 3 minutes. Remove the pot from the heat, cover and allow it to sit for 1 to 4 hours.

Boiling

After soaking and rinsing, fill a large pot to accommodate your beans or legumes with an excess of 1 inch of water. Lower the heat to reach a medium boil. Partially cover the pot with a lid. Cooking times vary according to the kind of bean or legume used and are shown below.

Rinsing

After soaking, drain the water from the pot and rinse the beans or legumes once or twice with fresh, cool water. This will wash off the indigestible sugars and anti-nutrients.

(Per 1 cup)	Soak Time	Cooking Time	Yield (in cups)
Azuki Beans	4 hrs.	45-55 min.	3
Anasazi Beans	4-8 hrs.	60 min.	2-1/4
Black Beans	4 hrs.	60-90 min.	2-1/4
Black-eyed Peas	-	60 min.	2
Cannellini Beans	8-12 hrs.	60 min.	2
Fava Beans	8-12 hrs.	40-50 min.	1-2/3
Chickpeas	6-8 hrs.	1-3 hrs.	2
Great Northern Beans	8-12 hrs.	1- 1/2 hrs.	2-2/3
Green Split Peas	-	45 min.	2
Yellow Split Peas	-	60-90 min.	2
Green Peas, whole	8-12 hrs.	1-2 hrs.	2
Kidney Beans	6-8 hrs.	60 min.	2-1/4
Lentils, brown	8-12 hrs.	45-60 min.	2-1/4
Lentils, green	8-12 hrs.	30-45 min.	2
Lentils, red or yellow	8-12 hrs.	20-30 min.	2 to 2-1/2
Lima Beans (large)	8-12 hrs.	45-60 min.	2
Lima Beans (small1	8-12 hrs.	50-60 min.	3
Mung Beans	-	60 min.	2
Navy Beans	6-8 hrs.	45-60 min.	2-2/3
Pink Beans	4-8 hrs.	50-60 min.	2-3/4
Pinto Beans	6-8 hrs.	1-1/2	2-2/3

Apple Sauce

Serves: 4 | Prep Time: ~40 minutes |

WHAT YOU NEED:

- 4 Jazz apples (peeled, cored, and quartered)

- 4 Red Delicious apples (peeled, cored, and quartered)

- ½ cup water

- 1 pinch Himalayan salt

- ½ tsp. cinnamon (optional)

- 1 tbsp. lemon juice (optional)

Total number of what you need: 6

HOW YOU MAKE IT:

1.   Put the apples into cold water for about 5 minutes.

2.   Remove the apples from the water and further cut the quarters into slices.

3.   Cook the slices of apple in a saucepan over medium heat with the water and salt.

4.   Stir often and bring down to a simmer after it starts to cook.

5.   After about 10 minutes of cooking, mash the apples while they are still simmering to create a sauce. Continue stirring and mashing further for about 20 minutes until you have a chunky apple

sauce.

6.   Add optional cinnamon and/or lemon juice if preferred.

7.   Let it cool.

8.   Blend if you prefer a smoother apple sauce.

Peanut Butter

Serves: 2 cups of peanut butter / 10 servings | Prep Time: ~15 minutes |

WHAT YOU NEED:

- 2 cups raw peanuts (unsalted)
- ½ tsp. Himalayan salt

Total number of what you need: 2

HOW YOU MAKE IT:

1. Preheat the oven to 375°F or 190°C.

2. Roast the peanuts for about 10 minutes.

3. Transfer them to a food processor and process for about 1 minute.

4. Scrape down the sides of the food processor, add the sea salt, and blend again for 1 minute; continue until the desired consistency is reached.

5. For the best flavor, chill the mix before serving.

Almond Milk

Serves: 5 | Prepping Time: 60 min |

WHAT YOU NEED:

1 cup raw almonds.

5 cups filtered water.

2 medjool dates, pitted.

1 teaspoon ground vanilla

1 pinch Himalayan salt.

Total number of what you need: 2

How you make it:

Grab a medium bowl, fill it with tap water and mix a pinch of salt with the water.

Place almonds in bowl, make sure that they're covered with water, and soak almonds overnight or for about 12 hours.

Remove almonds from salt mixture and rinse almonds in cold tap water.

Preheat oven on lowest setting.

Place rinsed almonds on a baking pan and put in oven to dry, check occasionally to see if the almonds are dry.

Once dry, remove almonds from oven and rinse again under cold water.

Pour the filtered water and almonds into a blender container.

Blend until it is creamy and smooth then strain mixture to filter out the leftover almond pulp.

Place the mixture back in blender and add the ground vanilla and the dates to mixture.

Blend until your preferred milk consistency is reached

Greenprint Breakfast Oat

Serves: 1 | Prep Time: ~15 min |

WHAT YOU NEED:

- 1 cup coconut milk

- ½ cup rolled oats

- 1 banana (medium, sliced)

- 4 cup blueberries (fresh or frozen)

- ½ tsp. vanilla extract (optional)

- 1 ½ tsp. agave syrup (optional) Toppings:

- 4 cup walnuts

- 4 cup raspberries (fresh or frozen)

- 1 tsp. chia seeds

Total number of what you need: 9

HOW YOU MAKE IT:

1. Combine the coconut milk, oats, banana and blueberries in a blender.

2. Add the optional vanilla and agave syrup.

3. Blend until smooth.

4. Pour into bowl.

5. Add the toppings and enjoy!

Berry-Bana Smoothie Bag

Serves: 1 | Prep Time: ~ 5 min |

WHAT YOU NEED:

- 1 cup blueberries (fresh or frozen)
- 1 cup raspberries (fresh or frozen)
- 1 cup strawberries (fresh or frozen)
- 1 cup blackberries (fresh or frozen)
- 2 bananas (medium, sliced)
- 2 green apples (skinned, cored, cubed)
- 2 cups water

Total number of what you need: 6

HOW YOU MAKE IT:

Place all the ingredients except the water in a freezer-friendly Ziploc bag and then place this in the freezer.

When you are ready to make the smoothie, pour about 2 cups of water into the blender followed by the smoothie bag ingredients and blend well.

Serve and enjoy!

Delicious Matcha Morning

Serves: 1 | Prep Time: ~15 min |

WHAT YOU NEED:

- 1 cup coconut milk

- 1 orange (skinned, parted)

- 1 cup kale (chopped)

- 1 banana (medium, sliced)

- ½ cup blueberries (fresh or frozen)

- 1 tsp. matcha powder

Toppings:

- ¼ cup pecans

- ¼ cup raspberries (fresh or frozen)

- 1 tsp. hemp seeds

Total number of what you need: 9

HOW YOU MAKE IT:

1. Combine the coconut milk, orange, kale, banana and blueberries in a blender.

2. Add the matcha powder.

3. Blend until smooth.

4. Pour the smoothie into a bowl.

5. Add toppings as you like and enjoy!

Powerhouse Protein Shake

Serves: 2 | Prep Time: ~5 min |

WHAT YOU NEED:

- 2 green apples (peeled, cored, and chopped)

- 1 cup pineapple chunks (fresh or frozen)

- 1 cup kale (fresh, chopped)

- 1 cup spinach (drained and rinsed)

- 1 tsp. spirulina

- 1 cup coconut water (alternatively use 3-4 ice cubes)

- 2 scoops of pea protein powder

Total number of what you need: 7

HOW YOU MAKE IT:

1. Add all the required ingredients to a blender.

2. Blend for 2 minutes.

3. Transfer to a large cup or shaker.

4. Enjoy!

Mango Blaster Smoothie Bag

Serves: 1 | Prep Time: ~ 5 min |

WHAT YOU NEED:

- 1 cup mango (chopped)

- 1 cup papaya (cubed)

- 1 cup blackberries (fresh or frozen)

- 2 bananas (medium, sliced)

- 1 cup coconut milk

- ½ cup water

Total number of what you need: 5

HOW YOU MAKE IT:

1.   Place all the ingredients except the coconut milk and water, in a freezer-friendly Ziploc bag and place in the freezer.

2.   When you are ready to make the smoothie, pour the coconut milk and V cup of water into the blender followed by the bag's ingredients and blend well.

3.   Serve and enjoy!

Peachy Mango Bowl

Serves: 1 | Prep Time: ~15 min |

WHAT YOU NEED:

- 1 peach (pitted, sliced)

- 1 mango (peeled, diced)

- 1 cup coconut milk

- 1 orange (skinned, parted)

- ¼ cup flaxseed (soaked)

- ½ cup pineapple chunks

Toppings:

- ¼ cup blueberries (fresh or frozen)

- ¼ cup pecans

- ¼ cup shredded coconut

Total number of what you need: 9

HOW YOU MAKE IT:

1. Add all the ingredients except the toppings to a blender.

2. Blend until smooth. Add water if necessary to reach the desired consistency.

3. Give it a good stir and pour the mixture into a bowl.

4. Add toppings as you like and enjoy!

Main Dishes

Here are some delicious lunch and dinner recipes for vegan families. There is variety in the ingredients, to give you the nutrition that you need. These dishes are relatively easy to make too, giving you more time with your family.

Vegetable Broth

Serves: 5 cups | Prep Time: ~90 min |

WHAT YOU NEED:

- 10 cups water
- 2 onions (chopped)
- 3 medium garlic cloves (minced)
- 4 carrots (chopped)
- 3 leafless celery ribs (chopped)
- 1 sweet potato (cubed)
- 1 red bell pepper (sliced)
- 1 cup fresh kale (or frozen, cut)
- ½ cup fresh parsley
- 1 tbsp. thyme (dried)
- 1 tbsp. rosemary (dried)
- Himalayan salt and black pepper to taste

Total number of what you need: 16

HOW YOU MAKE IT:

1. Preheat oven to 400°F / 200°C.

2. Put the onions, garlic, carrots, celery, sweet potato, bell pepper, kale, and parsley on an oven-proof roasting pan or baking tray.

3. Bake the veggies in the oven for about 20 minutes until browned and caramelized.

4. Put a large pot over medium heat and boil the water.

5. Add all ingredients from the roasting pan to the pot with boiling water.

6. Immediately bring the heat down to low and keep it at boiling point.

7. Stir every few minutes and add the miso paste, the optional nutritional yeast if desired, thyme, and rosemary.

8. Add salt, pepper, and any other desired spices to taste.

9.   Cook until half of the water has evaporated.

10.   Take the pot off the stove and let it cool.

11.   Pour the mixture through a sieve and collect the broth in a second pot. Don't waste the veggies afterwards; they make for a nice side dish!

12.   Use broth immediately, or store.

Tortilla Wraps

Serves: 8 | Prep Time: ~30 minutes |

WHAT YOU NEED:

- 2 ½ cups whole grain flour

- 2 tbsp. ground flaxseed

- ½ cup water

- Pinch of salt

Total number of what you need: 4

HOW YOU MAKE IT:

1. Add the flaxseed, the water, and salt to a medium bowl and mix well.

2. Let the bowl with the water and flaxseed sit for about 10 minutes before continuing.

3. Pour 2 cups of flour into the bowl and mix until dough forms.

4. Add more water if the dough is too dry to mold and falls apart.

5. Make a big ball of dough and split into 8 equal parts.

6. Sprinkle a bit of flour on a flat surface for every ball.

7. Flatten the ball with your hands, and sprinkle flour on the ball of dough when it gets too sticky.

8. Use a dough roller to flatten the ball into a thin circle. Spin the dough often to prevent it from sticking to the surface.

9. Make sure that your tortilla wrap is thin and about the size of a medium plate.

10. Put a large pan over high heat and cook the tortilla for about 30 seconds.

11. Repeat the process for the remaining balls to make 8 delicious tortillas.

Black Bean Soup

Serves: 4 | Prep Time: ~25 min |

WHAT YOU NEED:

- 2 cups dry black beans

- 2 cups water

- 4 cup green onions (chopped)

- 4 cup white onions (chopped)

- ½ cup chopped mushrooms

- 4 garlic cloves (chopped)

- ½ cup red bell peppers (chopped)

- 2 tsp. chili powder

- 2 tsp. ground cumin seeds

- Himalayan salt to taste

- Handful fresh parsley (optional, chopped)

Total number of what you need: 13

HOW YOU MAKE IT:

1. Prepare the black beans according to the method.

2. Transfer the cooked beans to a food processor or blender and add 1 cup of water.

3. Blend until the mixture is firm and smooth. Add more water if needed.

4. Put a medium-sized non-stick frying pan over medium heat.

5. Add the onions, mushrooms, garlic and red bell pepper.

6. Heat the vegetables for about 3 minutes while stirring and add the bean mixture with 1 cup of water.

7. Add more water, depending on the desired thickness.

8. Stir in the salt, chili powder and cumin seeds.

9. Turn the heat down to low and allow the soup to softly cook for 15 minutes, covered.

10. Serve with the optional fresh parsley on top.

11. Enjoy or store!

One Pan Ratatouille

The one-pan ratatouille is a vegetable stew that can be served over pasta or whole wheat bread, to make the main dish. It can also be served as a side dish with vegetable burgers. This dish is easy to make and contains a lot of vegetables that are good for your family's health.

Ingredients

- 8 ounces Asian eggplant, rinsed and diced
- 3 tbsps. olive oil
- 2 cans (14 1/2 oz. each) diced tomatoes
- 1 onion, peeled and diced
- 1 pound red, yellow, and/or orange bell peppers, de- seeded and diced
- 8 ounces yellow summer squash, diced
- 8 ounces zucchini, diced
- 3/4 cup chopped fresh basil leaves
- 2 cloves garlic, peeled and minced
- About 1/2 tsp. salt
- About 1/4 tsp. pepper

Method

1. Place a frying pan on medium heat and add 1 ½ tbsps.olive oil.
2. Add the garlic and onion and cook until the onion turns stiff.
3. Add the egg plant, tomatoes, pepper and water and bring to a simmer.
4. Cover and cook until the eggplant becomes soft.
5. Stir in the bell pepper, zucchini and squash and bring to a simmer and cover and cook until the squash becomes tender.
6. Add the remaining olive oil, stir in the basil leaves and garnish with salt and pepper.
7. Serve over pasta or whole wheat bread.

Yield: 4 servings

Five- Grain Cereal with Apples, Bananas and Apricots

This dish combines the wholesomeness of five grains with the goodness of fruits. This will be a full, wholesome breakfast or dinner dish for your family. The dry cereal can be stored in the refrigerator in a zip-up bag and you can cook up a nutritious meal for your family anytime.

Ingredients

- 1/2 cup oat bran
- 1/3 cup wheat bran
- 1/2 cup uncooked regular grits
- 1/3 cup flaxseed
- 1/2 cup cracked wheat
- 1 1/4 cups steel-cut (Irish) oats
- 2/3 cup dried apple, coarsely chopped
- 13 1/2 cups water
- 2/3 cup dried apricots, coarsely chopped
- 2/3 cup dried banana chips
- 3/4 tsp. salt

Method

1. Take a spice or coffee grinder and add the flaxseeds.
2. Grind it coarsely and pour it into a bowl.
3. Add all the other ingredients except water and mix well.
4. Boil water in a sauce pan and stir in the cereal.
5. Cover with a lid and cook over low heat for 15 minutes.
6. Ensure that you stir the mixture occasionally.
7. Uncover and cook for 2 more minutes.
8. Let it cool for a while and serve

Pan Crisped Tofu with Greens and Peanut Dressing

Tofu is a super food that is rich in proteins and calcium. Peanut is also rich in proteins and leafy greens are excellent for health. This dish is a healthy meal that you can cook up for your family as a lunch or dinner dish.

Ingredients

- 2 (14-ounce) packages of drained tofu
- 1/3 cup white miso (soybean paste)
- 1/3 cup mirin (sweet rice wine)
- 1/2 cup chopped dry-roasted peanuts, halved
- 5 tbsps. canola oil, divided
- 1/3 cup rice vinegar
- 8 cups gourmet salad greens
- 1 tbsp. of grated fresh ginger
- Minced fresh chives

Method

1. Mix the soybean paste, rice wine, vinegar, ginger, 1/4 cup peanuts and 3 tbsps. of oil in a bowl.
2. Cut each tofu block crosswise into 8 slices of ½ an inch.
3. Arrange the tofu pieces over paper towels, cover it with more layers of paper towels and place a heavy skillet on top to make it firm.
4. Wait for about 20 minutes before you remove the paper towels.
5. Place a large skillet over medium heat and 1 tbsp. of oil.
6. Add the 8 tofu slices. Sauté each side of the tofu pieces until it turns crisp.
7. Remove the tofu pieces and drain it with the paper towels.
8. Repeat this process with the remaining oil and the remaining 8 tofu pieces.
9. Take 8 plates and place 1 cup of greens in each.
10. Place 2 tofu slices over the greens and top it with 3 tbsps. of soybean paste ½ teaspoons of chopped peanuts.
11. Garnish with chives and serve.

Yield

8 servings

Vegetable Tagine with Baked Tempe

Tempe is a traditional soy product from Indonesia. It is rated as one of the healthiest foods in the world. It contains 38% of protein and is a rich source of iron and calcium. It is very good for growing children and teenagers. This dish has a Moroccan flavor to it. Your family will enjoy the delicious spiciness of this dish. You can make it less spicy for the children. You can serve this for lunch or dinner. Since this dish requires so many ingredients, you could reserve this dish for special days.

Ingredients

Tangine

- 1 cup zucchini (finely chopped)
- 1 cup peeled tomato (finely chopped)
- 1 cup yellow squash (finely chopped)
- 2 cups onion (finely chopped)
- 3/4 cup carrot (finely chopped)
- 2 cups (1/2-inch) cubed peeled sweet potato
- 2 cups chopped green cabbage
- 1 tsp. cumin seeds
- 1 tsp. caraway seeds
- 1 tsp. coriander seeds
- 1/2 tsp. paprika
- 1/2 tsp. black peppercorns
- 1 (1-inch) piece cinnamon stick
- 2 tsp. extra-virgin olive oil
- 1/2 cup celery (finely chopped)
- 1/2 tsp. sea salt
- 2 garlic cloves, peeled
- 1 1/2 cups water
- 1 tbsp. fresh lemon juice

Tempeh

- 1 pound tempeh, cut into 1/2-inch cubes
- 1/3 cup of chopped, fresh parsley
- 2 tsp ground cumin
- 6 tbsp. fresh lemon juice
- 2 tsp paprika
- 1/2 tsp ground red pepper
- 4 garlic cloves, minced
- 1/2 tsp sea salt
- 2/3 cup water

Remaining ingredients:

- 2 cups hot cooked couscous
- 4 tsp. minced fresh cilantro

Method

Tagine

1. Mix the cumin seeds, caraway seeds, coriander seeds, paprika, peppercorn and cinnamon sticks in a coffee grinder and process it until finely ground.
2. Place a skillet over medium heat and add the onion, carrot, celery, garlic and salt and cook for a few minutes while stirring.
3. Cover with a lid, reduce the heat and cook for about 20 minutes.
4. Stir in the spices mixture, sweet potato, cabbage, squash, zucchini, tomato and water and bring to a boil.
5. Reduce the heat and simmer it for 30 minutes until thick. Stir in the lemon juice.

Tempe

1. Pre-heat your oven to 350F.Mix the water, lemon juice, parsley, cumin, paprika, sea salt, red pepper and garlic in a pan.
2. Add the tempeh cubes and mix well until coated uniformly.
3. Arrange the tempeh mixture at the bottom of a baking dish and cover it with foil.
4. Place it in the oven and bake it at 35minutes.
5. Uncover and bake until the liquid is completely absorbed.
6. Serve tempeh over tagine and couscous, garnished with cilantro.

Yield

4   Servings

Quinoa Tabbouleh

Quinoa has often been called the super grain of the millennium. It contains a high amount of dietary fiber and high quality proteins similar to those found in meat. Quinoa can be a meat substitute for vegan families. Tabbouleah is an Arab salad. You can combine various ingredients according to your family's choice. Quinoa Tabbouleh is an easy dinner/lunch recipe that you can cook up for your family.

Ingredients

- 1 cup uncooked quinoa
- 1 3/4 cups water
- 1/2 cup chopped tomato
- 1/4 cup chopped cucumber
- 2 tbsps. chopped green onions
- 1/2 cup chopped fresh mint or parsley
- 1/4 cup raisins
- 1/4 cup fresh lemon juice
- 2 tsp. minced fresh onion
- 1 tbsp. extra-virgin olive oil
- 1/2 tsp. salt
- 1/4 tsp. of ground black pepper

Method

1. Take a sauce pan and add the water and quinoa to it.
2. Bring it to a boil.
3. Cover it and simmer for 20 minutes until the water is completely absorbed.
4. Remove from the heat and stir it well.
5. Add all the remaining ingredients and mix well.
6. Cover and wait for an hour. Serve chilled or at room temperature.

Yield

5 servings

Potato Curry with Roti or Rice

This potato curry is of Caribbean parentage and made with potato and acorn squash. There is a mild sweetness to this dish which your family will enjoy. They also get a good amount of vegetables from this dish. It can be served with rice or stuffed inside the Indian flatbread called Roti. This can be a lunch or dinner dish.

Ingredients

- 4 cups (1-inch) cubed peeled Yukon gold potato
- 3 cups (1-inch) cubed peeled acorn squash
- 1 1/2 cups chopped onion
- 1 cup chopped red bell pepper
- 1 1/4 tsp. salt
- 2 tsp. ground cumin
- 1 1/2 tsp. ground turmeric
- 1 tsp. ground ginger
- 1/4 tsp. ground allspice
- 1/4 tsp. crushed red pepper
- 1 tbsp. canola oil
- 4 garlic cloves, minced
- 1/2 cup light coconut milk
- 1/2 cup chopped fresh cilantro
- 2 cups water

Method

1. Mix the salt, cumin, turmeric, ginger, allspice and red pepper and keep it aside.
2. Place a skillet over medium heat and add the onions.
3. Cook it until tender, stirring constantly.
4. Add garlic and cook for about 15 seconds.
5. Add spice mixture and cook for about 30 seconds.
6. Add potato squash and bell pepper and stir well to mix it with the spices.
7. Cook for about a minute. Stir in the water and coconut milk and bring it to a boil.
8. Cover the skillet and reduce the heat. Let it simmer until the potato is tender. Garnish with cilantro.
9. Serve it with rice or roti.

Yield

6   Servings

Koshari

Koshari is an Egyptian dish that is rich in starch. It contains rice, pasta and legumes and is topped with spicy-sweet tomatoes and caramelized onions. This dish can take care of the carbohydrate requirements of your family, providing them with oodles of energy. You can serve this as lunch or dinner.

Ingredients

Sauce

- 2 (14.5-ounce) cans diced tomatoes, undrained
- 1 cup finely chopped onion
- 1 tbsp. extra-virgin olive oil
- 1 1/2 tbsps. minced garlic
- 1/2 tsp. crushed red pepper
- 1/2 tsp. sea salt
- 1/2 tsp. of ground black pepper

Koshari

- 1 1/4 cups of dried lentils
- 2 1/2 cups of hot cooked long-grain rice
- 3 cups thinly sliced onion
- 1/2 cup of uncooked vermicelli, broken into 1-inch pieces
- 3 tbsps. extra-virgin olive oil
- 5 cups water
- 1 tsp. sea salt

Method

Sauce

1. Take a skillet and place it over medium heat.
2. Add 1 tbsp. of oil and the onions.
3. Cook for 15 minutes until golden.
4. Add the garlic and cook for 2 minutes.
5. Add ½ tsp. salt, pepper and tomatoes.
6. Cook for 10 minutes until it becomes slightly thick.
7. Transfer this tomato mix to a blender and blend until smooth. Keep it warm.

Koshari

1. Place a skillet over medium heat and add 3 tbsps. Of oil to it.
2. Add onions and cook until golden brown.
3. Remove the onions and set it aside.

4. Add vermicelli to the skillet and sauté until golden brown. Remove from the heat and keep it aside.
5. Keep a sauce pan over medium heat and add water and lentil. Bring it to a boil.
6. Cover it, reduce the heat and let it simmer for 30 minutes until the lentils become tender.
7. Remove from the heat and add the vermicelli to it and cover the mouth of the pan with a kitchen towel. Let it remain for 10 minutes until the vermicelli is tender.
8. Add rice and 1 tsp. salt to the lentil-vermicelli mixture. Mix well with a fork and serve with sauce and onions.

Yield

4 Servings

Seitan Stir fry with Black Bean Garlic Sauce

Seitan, also known as wheat gluten is a vegetarian meat substitute made from wheat, soy sauce, ginger, garlic and seaweed. It is a powerhouse of proteins and iron and is low in fat. Black bean contains protein, fiber, micronutrients and antioxidants. This meal can be a protein-rich lunch and dinner dish for your family.

Ingredients

- 2 cups thinly sliced drained seitan
- 1 ounce dried shiitake mushrooms
- 2 tbsps. of Chinese rice wine
- 4 cups (2-inch) cut green beans
- 2 cups hot cooked brown rice
- 2 cups boiling water
- 2 tbsps. black bean garlic sauce 2 tsp. cornstarch
- 2 tbsps. canola oil, divided
- 1 tbsp. finely chopped garlic
- 1 tbsp. of chopped, fresh ginger
- 1/4 tsp. salt
- Cilantro sprigs

Method

1. Boil 2 cups of water in a bowl and add mushrooms to the boiling water.
2. Cover and let it remain for 20 minutes. Set aside ½ cup of the soaking liquid and drain the rest in a colander over a bowl.
3. Drain the mushrooms well and remove the stems.
4. Thinly slice the mushroom caps. Mix the ½ cup soaking liquid, corn starch, rice wine and black bean sauce and set it aside.
5. Place a skillet on medium heat and add 1 tbsp. of canola oil .Add the seitan and stir-fry until golden brown.
6. Remove the seitan and place it in a bowl. Heat the remaining 1 tbsp. oil in the same skillet and add ginger and garlic and stir fry for 30 seconds.
7. Add beans and mushrooms and cover and cook for 3 minutes. Add black bean sauce.
8. Cook until the sauce becomes thick. Add seitan to the pan and cook for a minute. Remove from heat.
9. Garnish with cilantro and serve over rice.

Yield

4   servings

Barbecued Tempe Sandwiches with Peppers and Onion

Tempeh is a soy product that is rich in proteins is very similar to a burger patty. It has a nutty flavor that goes well with the sweet and spicy barbeque sauce to give a taste that your family will love.

Ingredients

- 1 (8-ounce) package tempeh
- 4 (1 1/2-ounce) hamburger buns
- 1 red onion, cut into 1/2-inch-thick slices
- 1 red bell pepper, cut in half
- 1 yellow bell pepper, cut in half
- 1/3 cup ketchup
- 1 tbsp. brown sugar
- 1 1/2 tsp. vegetable oil
- 1 1/2 tsp. cider vinegar
- 1 tsp. Dijon mustard
- 1/4 tsp. chili powder
- 1/4 tsp. low-sodium soy sauce
- 1/4 tsp. hot sauce
- 1 garlic clove, minced
- Cooking spray

Method

Prepare the grill

1. Mix the ketchup, brown sugar, oil, vinegar, mustard, chili powder, soy and hot sauces and garlic in a bowl.
2. Cut tempe in half, lengthwise and cut the slices in half. Brush tempe slices, bell peppers and onions with the ketchup mix.
3. Place the tempe slices on the grill coated with cooking spray and grill each side for about 4 minutes.
4. Grill the bell peppers and onions too. Cut the bell peppers into ½ inch strips and separate the onions into rings.
5. Place a tempe slice on the bottom half of each bun. Top it with ¼ of bell pepper and ¼ of onions and close with the top half of the bun.

Yield

4 sandwiches

Easy Vegetable Paella

The Spanish Paella is healthy rice and provides the carbohydrates required by your body. It also contains Vitamins B1 and B2.Vegatable Paella will be good lunch or dinner choice for your family.

Ingredients

- 9oz (~250g) Risotto or Paella Rice
- ½ cup tomato puree
- 20oz (600ml) vegetable broth
- 1 medium Sweet Potato - peeled and diced 1 inch
- 1 medium Zucchini - peeled, chopped 1 inch
- 4 tbsps. Olive Oil
- 1 medium White Onion - diced into ½inch pieces
- 4 cloves of Garlic - crushed
- 1 Jalapeno
- 7oz canned Sweet Corn
- 10 small tomatoes - quartered
- 2 tbsps. of dried mixed herbs or ½cup of parsley or cilantro
- Lemon juice
- Salt and Pepper to taste

Method

1. Heat olive oil in a skillet and add onions and some salt to it.
2. Sauté until tender and then add garlic and jalapeño.
3. Sauté for a few more minutes and then add sweet potato, zucchini, tomatoes and corn and sauté for a few more minutes.
4. Stir in rice and tomato puree. Slowly add the vegetable broth without stirring. Top with herbs and pepper.
5. Cover and let it simmer for 20 minutes. Let all the liquid get absorbed.
6. Squeeze in the lemon juice and serve hot.

Easy Mexican Freekeh Pilaf

Freekeh is a whole grain made of young, toasted green wheat. It is a slow-release energy food and has many health benefits.

Ingredients

- 1 cup Freekeh (whole)
- 1 Tomato (diced)
- 2½ cups Vegetable Broth
- 1 tbsp. Olive Oil
- ½ yellow Onion (diced)
- 1 Zucchini (diced)
- 1 red Bell Pepper (diced)
- 1 cup Sweet Corn
- 1 cup Kidney Beans
- 1 tbsp. Chili Powder
- 1 tsp. Cumin
- 1 tsp. Oregano
- 1 tsp. Garlic Powder
- 2 tsp. Paprika
- 1handful fresh Cilantro (roughly chopped)
- 1 Jalapeno
- Lime Juice
- ½ tsp. ground Black Pepper

Method

1. Place a sauce pan on medium heat.
2. Add olive oil and onion and sauté until soft.
3. Add zucchini and bell pepper and sauté for a few more minutes.
4. Add corn, tomato, beans, freekeh, herbs, spices and half the cilantro.
5. Mix well in the pan .Add the vegetable broth and bring to a boil.
6. Let it simmer over reduced heat for about 40 minutes.
7. Garnish with jalapeno and cilantro and a sprinkle of lime juice and serve hot.

Yield

4   Servings

Tempeh Rendang

This is a Malaysian stew that is full of flavor. The tempeh soaks in the flavor of the herbs and the sweetness of coconut milk. You can serve it with steamed rice for lunch or dinner.

Ingredients

- 1 1/2 pounds tempeh, cut into 1/2-inch cubes
- 1 cup light coconut milk
- 1 cup minced shallots (about 6)
- 1 1/2 tbsps. of grated, fresh galangal
- 1/3 cup of shredded unsweetened coconut, toasted.
- 1 tsp. of kosher salt
- 6 red Thai chilies, thinly sliced
- Cooking spray
- 1 tbsp. of grated ginger
- 1 tbsp. of chopped fresh lemongrass (about 1 stalk)
- 1/4 tsp. ground turmeric
- 1/2 cup water
- 2 kaffir lime leaves
- 2 tbsps. chopped fresh cilantro

Method

1. Place a skillet over medium heat and coat with cooking spray.
2. Add chilies, shallots, galangal, ginger, lemongrass and turmeric and cook for 5 minutes until fragrant.
3. Add coconut milk, lime leaves, ½ cup water, salt and tempeh to the pan.
4. Cover and simmer it over reduced heat until the sauce thickens. Remove the lime leaves.
5. Garnish with the remaining cilantro and coconut. Serve with rice.

Yield

5 servings

Peanut Sauce Stir fry with Tempeh

This dish provides a double dose of proteins to your family, combining tempeh with peanut sauce. The nutty taste makes this popular among children and adults alike. Can be served over rice.

Ingredients

- 8 ounces Tempeh (diced)
- 2 tbsps. Olive Oil
- 2 cups Rice
- 1 cup Vegetable Broth
- 2 carrots (sliced)
- 1 cup Bamboo Shoot Strips
- 1 small yellow Onion (diced)
- 1 yellow Bell Pepper
- 1 tsp. fresh Ginger (finely diced)
- 2 cloves of Garlic (crushed)
- ⅓ cup Peanut Butter
- 3 tbsps. Soy Sauce
- 3 tbsps. Pure Maple Syrup
- Red Pepper Flakes (optional)
- 1 handful chopped Peanuts (optional)

Method

1. Prepare the rice as per the instructions.
2. Place a small frying pan over medium heat and add olive oil.
3. Fry both sides of the tempeh until browned.
4. Mix the vegetable broth, peanut butter, soy sauce and maple syrup in a bowl and whisk it well to make the peanut sauce.
5. Add 1 tbsp. olive oil to a big pan and add onion, carrots, bell pepper, ginger and garlic.
6. Stir fry over medium heat for about 10 minutes. Add tempeh, bamboo shoots, and the peanut sauce.
7. Continue frying until the sauce thickens. Serve as a side dish with rice.

Yield:

4 Servings

Moroccan Flatbreads

Moroccan flatbreads paired with vegan feta cheese salad, bell pepper and bell pepper will give you a wonderful North African meal. This can be a special meal for your family, special occasions. These flat breads stuffed with vegetables and are a treat to your taste buds.

Ingredients

- 1/2 tsp. dry yeast
- 2 cups chopped onion
- 1/2 cup finely chopped fresh flat-leaf parsley
- 3/4 cup plus 1 tbsp. warm water (100° to 110°)
- 9 ounces all-purpose flour (about 2 cups)
- 3/4 tsp. sea salt
- 1/2 tsp. sea salt
- 1/4 tsp. crushed red pepper
- 2 tbsps. extra-virgin olive oil
- 2 tsp. paprika
- 1 tsp. ground cumin
- 1 tsp. canola oil, divided
- Cooking spray

Method

1. Take a large bowl of warm water and dissolve yeast in it. Keep it aside for 5 minutes.
2. Add flour and ¾ tsp. salt to the yeast mixture and stir it in with a wooden spoon.
3. Spread the dough on a lightly floured surface and knead with your hand for a few minutes to get a smooth texture.
4. Divide the dough into 8 equal portions and make 8 balls with it. Lightly coat with the cooking spray, cover with a plastic wrap and wait for 30 minutes.
5. Mix the onions, paprika, parsley, olive oil, cumin, sea salt and pepper in a bowl.
6. Flatten out each ball of dove into a 6 ½ inch circle. Spoon 2 tbsps. of the onion mixture in the center of the circle.
7. Cover up the filling by folding the sides over it. Press the sides gently to seal it. Repeat the process with all the dough balls.
8. Place a large non-stick skillet over medium heat and add ½ tsp. oil to it. Cook the flatbreads 4 at a time in the pan.
9. Cook each side of the bread for 2 minutes. Repeat the procedure for the remaining 4 flatbreads.

Yield

8 flatbreads

Tofu Banh Mi

This is sandwich with a Vietnamese flavor. The tofu is marinated, soaking up the spicy zing of ginger and the savory flavor of soya sauce.

Ingredients

- 1(14-ounce) package water-packed firm tofu, drained
- 1 1/4 cups (3-inch) matchstick-cut carrot
- 1 julienne-cut green onion
- 1 cup sliced shiitake mushroom caps
- 1/3 cup rice vinegar
- 2 tbsps. low-sodium soy sauce
- 2 tsp. finely grated peeled fresh ginger
- 1/4 cup sugar
- 1tsp. kosher salt
- 1/4 tsp. freshly ground black pepper
- 1 cucumber, peeled, halved lengthwise, and thinly sliced (about 2 cups)
- 2 tbsps. canola oil
- 2 jalapeño peppers, thinly sliced
- 1 (12-ounce) loaf French bread
- 1/2 cup fresh cilantro sprigs

Method

1. Cut tofu crosswise to form 8 half inch slices. Place tofu on several layers of paper towels and cover with more paper towels.
2. Top it with a heavy pan and let it stand for half an hour.
3. Take a baking dish and mix the soy sauce and ginger in it Arrange the tofu slices in a single layer in this mixture.
4. Cover and keep in the refrigerator for about 8 hours. Take a medium bowl and mix the sugar, vinegar and salt and stir well to dissolve the sugar and salt.
5. Add carrot, mushroom, cucumber and onion and mix well. Let it remain for 30 minutes.
6. Drain the carrot mixture thoroughly.
7. Place a skillet over medium heat and add oil. Remove the tofu slices from the marinade and pat it dry with paper towels.
8. Sauté the tofu slices in the pan until both sides are browned.
9. Preheat broiler. Cut bread in half lengthwise and arrange it on a baking dish, cut side up.
10. Broil until it turns lightly brown. Place the tofu slices on the bottom half of the bread and top it with carrot mixture, jalapeno slices and cilantro.
11. Close it with top half. Cut the loaf into 6 pieces and serve.

Yield

6 sandwiches

Pizzas and Pastas

Pizzas and pastas are a favorite among younger and older people in the family. Here are some pizza and pasta recipes that are simply amazing

Cilantro Basil Pesto Pasta

Pesto with pasta is a winning combination and your family will love it. Opt for gluten free pasta or whole wheat pasta.

Ingredients

- 4 cups Farfalle Whole Wheat Pasta(cooked)
- ½ cup raw, unsalted Cashews
- ¼ to ½ tsp. fresh Ginger
- ½ cup Olive Oil
- ½ cup fresh Basil
- 1 cup fresh Cilantro
- 1 large Garlic clove
- ½ tsp. Lemon Juice
- Fresh Cracked Pepper
- ¼ tsp. Salt

Method
1. Blend all ingredients except the pasta in a blender until smooth.
2. Mix the pesto with the hot pasta and serve, garnished with fresh cracked pepper.

Yield

4   Servings

Coconut and Garlic White Pizza

This an interesting take on the conventional white pizza. The ingredients are interesting and the pizza is savory.

Ingredients

- Pizza Dough
- Pizza Topping
- 2 cups (250g) Whole Wheat Flour
- ½ a cube of Fresh Active Yeast (0.30ounces or 8g)
- ½ cup Water (warm)
- 1 medium sized Shallot or Red Onion (diced, or in small rings)
- ½ Red Bell Pepper (finely diced)
- ¾ tsp. Salt
- 1 tsp. Whole Cane Sugar
- Coconut Garlic Sauce
- ½ cup full fat Coconut Milk
- Cloves of Garlic (crushed)
- 2 tsp. Olive Oil
- 1 tsp. dried Oregano
- ½ tsp. Salt
- Fresh cracked Pepper (optional)

Method

1. Mix yeast, 2 tbsps. of flour and 1/2 cup warm water .Let it stand for 10 minutes.
2. Knead the dough with your hand until it is soft and moist and non-sticky.
3. Cover dough with a plastic wrap and let it remain in a warm place for about half an hour until it doubles in size.
4. Pre-heat oven to 450F.
5. Meanwhile place a skillet over medium heat and heat olive oil in it.
6. Add garlic and sauté for a few minutes Add coconut milk and salt and bring to a boil.
7. Reduce the heat and simmer for 3-5 minutes and set it aside.
8. Take half of the dough and using a rolling pin, roll it out into pizza crust.
9. Lay it out on a sheet pan lined with parchment paper and cover it to let it rise.
10. Do this with the remaining dough to form a second pizza crust.
11. Slowly add the coconut garlic sauce to the base. Top it with shallots, bell pepper and oregano.
12. Bake it in the oven for 10minutes.Garnish with pepper and serve

Yield

2 pizzas

Healthy Spinach Pine Nut Pizza

This dish is the best way to get the kids and teenagers in the family to eat their greens. Pine nuts are rich in vitamins, minerals, anti-oxidants and dietary fiber.

Ingredients

- 2 cups (250g) Whole Wheat Flour
- ½ Cup (125ml) Tomato Puree
- 1 medium sized Shallot or Red Onion (diced, or in small rings)
- 1 cup Baby Spinach (washed and dried)
- 2 tbsps. Pine Nuts
- ½ a cube of Fresh Active Yeast (0.30ounces or 8g) or 1 Packet Dry Yeast
- ¾ tsp. Salt
- 1 tsp. Whole Cane Sugar
- 1 tbsp. dried oregano
- 1 tbsp. dried basil
- Salt and crushed Pepper to taste
- 3 tbsps. Olive Oil
- ½ tsp. Salt
- Fresh cracked Pepper

Method

1. Combine the yeast, ½ cup water and 2 tbsps. of flour and let it remain for 10 minutes.
2. Knead with your hands until the dough becomes soft and moist.
3. Cover the dough with a plastic wrap and place in a warm place for 20-40 minutes until it doubles in size.
4. Preheat your oven to 450F.
5. To make the tomato sauce, mix the tomato puree, dried oregano, dried basil, salt and crushed pepper and keep it aside.
6. Take half the dough and using a rolling pin, roll each half into a pizza crust.
7. Take a baking dish and lay a parchment paper as lining. Keep the pizza base in the dish and cover the base with tomato sauce.
8. Top it with onions, spinach, pine nuts and salt. Sprinkle some olive oil and bake in the oven for 10 minutes.
9. Garnish with pepper and serve.

Yield

2 pizzas

Tempeh- Pasta Casserole

This is a protein-rich dish that can be easily put together for your family at dinner or lunch time. The pasta provides the carbohydrates that your family requires.

Ingredients

- 7 ounces (200g) Tempeh (diced)
- 3 cups Whole Wheat Shell Pasta (cooked)
- 6 medium Tomatoes (roughly diced)
- 1 medium White or Yellow Onion (diced)
- 1 tbsps. of Olive Oil
- 2 Garlic Cloves (crushed)
- 1 tbsp. of Fresh Rosemary
- 1 cup of whole Cashews, unsalted
- ¼ tsp. of Salt
- 1 tsp. of dried Oregano
- ½ cup Unsweetened Almond or Oat Milk
- 1 tsp. of White Wine Vinegar
- 1 tsp. Olive Oil
- ¼ tsp. of Salt
- ¼ tsp. of fresh cracked Pepper

Method

1. Place a stock pot over medium heat and add olive oil to it. Add diced onion and sauté until for a few minutes.
2. Add rosemary and garlic and sauté for a few more minutes until the tempe becomes light brown.
3. Add tomatoes, 1/4 tsp. salt and pepper into the stockpot and cover and cook for 10 minutes.
4. Pre-heat oven to 475F.
5. Blend cashews, ¼ tsp. salt and oregano in a blender to make thick, creamy cashew cheese. Keep it aside.
6. Add almond milk to the tomato mix in the stockpot and bring it to a boil.
7. Reduce the heat and let it simmer for a few minutes, until it thickens.
8. Stir in the cooked pasta and white vinegar to this mixture.
9. Pour into a baking dish and sprinkle with crumpled cashew cheese.
10. Sprinkle olive oil and bake in the oven for 5 minutes until the cashew cheese is browned.

Yield

5   Servings

Vegetable Arugula Whole Wheat Pizza

This is a delectable dish for the pizza lovers in the family. It combines the wholesomeness of whole grain with the goodness of sundried tomatoes.

Ingredients

- 1 Garlic Clove
- 8 Sundried Tomatoes (not in Olive Oil)
- ⅓ Cup (75ml) Olive Oil
- 6 Walnut halves
- ½ Cup (125ml) Tomato Puree
- 1 tbsp. of dried oregano
- 1 tbsp. of dried basil
- Salt and crushed Pepper to taste
- ½ Zucchini
- 1 Bell pepper (orange, red, or yellow)
- 4 tbsps. of sweet corn (canned)
- 2 tbsps. of Olive Oil
- Large handful of Arugula
- 1 Packet Dry Yeast 16oz (8.75g)
- 2 cups (250g) Whole Wheat Flour
- 1 tbsp. Salt
- 1/2cup warm water

Method

1. Mix the yeast, flour, water and salt and let it stand for 10 minutes.
2. Knead it with the hand until smooth and soft. Cover it with a plastic wrap and keep in a warm place.
3. Let it remain there for 20-40 minutes.
4. Blend the tomato puree, oregano, basil, salt and pepper in a blender to make the tomato sauce.
5. Wash the Zucchini and bell pepper and cut into thin slices. Rinse the corn. Mix these in a sauce pan.
6. Add olive oil and heat it for a few minutes. Wash and dry the Arugula. Mix it and keep it aside. This is the pizza topping.
7. Pre-heat the oven to 450F.
8. Take half the dough and using a rolling pin, roll each half into a pizza crust.
9. Take a baking dish and line it with parchment paper. Place the crust at the bottom of the dish and cover it with tomato sauce and spread the pizza topping uniformly on the top. Bake it in the oven for 10 minutes

Yield

2   Pizzas

Soups and Salads

Here are some Plant based soups and salads that you can quickly whip up for your family.

Easy Roasted Butternut Squash Soup

Nuts contain proteins and give an irresistible taste when added to any dish. Here is a soup that you can relish.

Ingredients

- 1 Butternut Squash(halved and seeded)
- 2 tsp. of Olive Oil
- 2 cups of Vegetable Broth
- 1 Large Onion
- 14 oz. can of Coconut milk
- 1 small Garlic head
- 1 tbsp. Curry Powder
- Salt and Pepper to taste
- Cayenne Pepper to taste

Method

1. Pre-heat oven to 350F.Line your pan with baking paper and place the quartered onions, squash brushed with oil and the garlic head wrapped in a foil.
2. Roast for 40-60 minutes. Once it cools down, take out the garlic head, cut the end and squeeze the pulp into a stockpot.
3. Scoop out the flesh from the butternut squash and place it in the stockpot.
4. Add the quartered onions. Add the vegetable broth and mix well.
5. Place the stockpot on medium heat and bring the contents to a boil.
6. Add coconut milk and spices, stirring constantly. Bring to a boil once again and then simmer over low heat for 10minutes.
7. Serve with toasted bread and pine nuts.

Yield

8   servings

Moroccan Red Gazpacho

This is a Moroccan soup that spicy and tangy and can make a great combination when served with pita bread.

- 1 (6 1/2-inch) pita, torn into pieces
- 4 large ripe plum tomatoes, coarsely chopped
- 1 large red bell pepper, seeded and coarsely chopped
- 1 large cucumber, peeled, seeded, and coarsely chopped
- 1/4 small yellow onion, chopped
- 1/2 cup boiling water
- 2 cups unsalted tomato puree
- 4 tbsps. extra-virgin olive oil, divided
- 2 tbsps. sherry vinegar
- 1 cup cold water
- 2 tsp. ras el hanout(spice blend from Morocco)
- 1/2 tsp. ground cumin
- 1/4 tsp. ground cinnamon
- 2 tbsps. chopped fresh cilantro
- 3/4 tsp. salt

Method

1. Take a bowl and add the pita bread. Pour the boiling water to cover it.
2. Let it stay for 1 minute. Drain and keep it aside. Blend the pita, 1 tbsp. oil, vinegar, tomatoes, bell pepper, cucumber and onion in a blender to get a smooth mix.
3. Place this mix in a bowl and stir in the tomato puree, the spice powder, cumin and cinnamon.
4. Cover and refrigerate for 2 hours. Ladle the soup into 8 bowls, top it with 1 tsp. oil and ¾ tsp. cilantro and serve.

Yield

8   Servings

Apple Beet Soup

Beets are a rich source of anti-oxidants for your family. Soups are a good way of including it in your diet.

Ingredients

- 1 tbsp. Olive Oil
- 1 small white or yellow Onion
- 1 large Beet (peeled, diced into 1/2 inch cubes)
- 1/4 tsp. Salt
- 1/2 sweet Apple (peeled, cored, diced)
- 2 cups Vegetable Broth
- 1 tsp. Lemon Juice
- Coconut Cream
- Parsley for garnish

Method

1. Take ½ the apples in a bowl and mix it with lemon juice and keep it aside.
2. Place a sauce pan over medium heat and add olive oil.
3. Add onions and salt and sauté until soft. Add the beets and the remaining apple.
4. Cook for 5 minutes while stirring. Add the vegetable broth and bring it to a boil. Simmer over low heat for 20 minutes.
5. Puree the soup in a blender and ladle it into bowls. Garnish with coconut cream, lemon, 1 tsp. of lemon-apple topping and fresh parsley.

Yield

4 servings

Red Lentil Carrot Soup

Lentils are rich in proteins, fibers and folates and can reduce cholesterol levels in the body. Carrot contains beta carotenes and has cancer-fighting and anti-ageing properties. This soup is an ideal health food for your family

Ingredients

- 1 cup uncooked Red Lentils (rinsed with cold water)
- 1½ cups grated Carrots
- 2 tbsps. Olive Oil
- 1 White Onion (finely diced)
- 2 tomatoes (diced)
- 1 tsp. grated fresh Ginger
- 2 cloves Garlic (minced)
- 4 tbsps. Red Curry Paste
- 1 Red Bell Pepper (diced)
- 4 cups Water
- 1 tbsp. Lime Juice
- ¾ cups Coconut Milk

Method

1. Place a stock pot over medium heat and add oil to it. Add the onion and ginger and cook for a few minutes.
2. Add garlic and red curry paste and cook for a few more minutes. Stir in the carrot, tomatoes and bell pepper.
3. Cover and cook for 5-10 minutes. Add lentils and water and bring to a boil. Simmer over reduced heat until the lentils become soft.
4. Pour the coconut milk and lime juice, stirring constantly. Bring to a cook boil and serve. Garnish with basil, whipped coconut cream or red chili flakes

Yield

9   servings

Asian Spring Vegetable Soup with Tofu

This is a delicious soup that gives your family the goodness of vegetables combined with the health benefits of tofu.

Ingredients

- 4 cups Vegetable Broth (I prefer organic, low sodium)
- 1 Red Bell Pepper (sliced)
- 1 Yellow Bell Pepper (sliced)
- 2 Carrots (peeled and julienned)
- 7 ounces organic Firm Tofu (diced)
- 3.50ounces Cellophane Noodles or Glass noodles
- 2 Scallions (sliced)
- 1 thumb sized piece of Fresh Ginger (sliced)
- 1 large Garlic Clove (sliced)
- 1 fresh Cayenne Pepper (chopped)
- 1 Lemongrass stalk
- Sugar Snap Peas
- 1 tbsp. Olive Oil
- Salt and Pepper

Method

1. Take a stock pot an d pour the vegetable broth into it. Add the ginger, garlic, cayenne pepper and lemongrass stalk and bring it to a boil.
2. Remove from the heat and let it cool for 15 minutes.
3. Cook the noodles according to directions.
4. Remove the lemongrass from the boiled broth and add sugar snap peas. Bring the broth to a boil once again and let it simmer for a few minutes.
5. Fry the tofu in olive oil for a few minutes and season it with salt and pepper. Add the tofu, cooked noodles, carrots, bell peppers and scallions to the broth.
6. Simmer for a few minutes. Serve hot.

Yield
4 servings

Antioxidant Cherry Fruit Salad

Cherries are well-known for their antioxidant properties. Here is a salad that is tasty and boosts your immune system. The kids will love the sweetness of cherry.

Ingredients

- 15 Bing Cherries (halved, pits removed)
- 20 Blueberries
- 1 Kiwi (peeled, halved and sliced)
- 1 tsp. Pistachios (chopped)

Method

1. Take a bowl and mix the cherries, blue berries and kiwi in a bowl.
2. Serve it with pistachios on top.

Yield

2 servings

Watermelon and Heirloom Tomato Salad

Watermelons are a powerful, body-healing fruit. Tomatoes are another super food that fights many diseases. This salad combines the two to give you a dish that is fortifying and tasty too.

Ingredients

- 12 Mini Heirloom Tomatoes (sliced)
- 1 cup diced Watermelon
- ¼ cup Fresh Dill (washed, chopped)
- 1 medium Red Onion (sliced)
- 1 Cucumber (sliced)
- Salt and Pepper to taste
- 1 Lemon

Method

1. Take a bowl and mix the tomatoes, watermelon, cucumber, onion and dill.
2. Cut the lemon and squeeze the juice over the salad. Garnish with salt and pepper and serve.

Yield

3   Servings

Beluga Black Lentil Salad with Rice

Black lentils are good source of proteins, vitamins, minerals and dietary fiber. This salad packs a healthy punch in your diet.

Ingredients

- ½ cup uncooked Rice (brown, wild, & red)
- ¼ cup uncooked Beluga or Black Lentils
- 1 scallion (ends removed, sliced)
- 1 Handful fresh Cilantro (chopped)
- 1 large Tomato (diced)
- ¼ cup Olive Oil
- 1 tbsp. Lemon Juice
- 1 Garlic Clove (crushed)
- 1 tsp. Paprika (ground)
- ½ tsp. Cumin (ground)
- ¼ tsp. Coriander (ground)
- ½ tsp. dried Marjoram
- pinch of Cayenne Pepper
- Salt and Pepper to taste

Method

1. Cook rice and lentils according to instructions. Take a bowl and add the spices, herbs, olive oil and lemon juice and whisk well.
2. Pour over the cooked and drained lentil and rice. Add tomatoes and scallions and mix all the ingredients well.
3. Add salt and pepper as per your taste.

Yield

4   servings

Vegan Pasta Salad with Lime

This is a salad that you can quickly put together for your family, that is filling and full of flavor.

Ingredients

- 16 ounces Whole Wheat Shell Pasta (cooked and drained)
- 25 small Plum Tomatoes (quartered)
- 1 cucumber (diced)
- 1 medium Red Onion (finely diced)
- ¾ cup low sodium Vegetable Broth
- ¼ cup Olive Oil
- 5 tbsps. fresh Lime Juice
- ½ cup fresh Cilantro (chopped)
- 5 tbsps. Apple Cider Vinegar
- 2 cups Corn
- Salt and pepper to taste

Method

1. Cook pasta as per instructions and drain well.
2. Add lime juice, olive oil, cilantro, vegetable broth and vinegar while it is warm and mix well. Let it cool.
3. Add the corn, tomatoes, onions and cucumber and mix well.
4. Add salt and pepper and top it with cilantro leaves.

Yield:

12 Servings

Mango Bean Salsa

Mango is a super fruit that contains 20 different kinds of vitamins and minerals. It contains glutamine acid that can improve concentration and memory. It is an aphrodisiac too!

Ingredients

- 1 Mango (diced)
- 8 small Tomatoes (cut into eights)
- ⅓ cup Kidney Beans
- ½ small Red Onion (finely diced)
- small handful of Cilantro (chopped)
- Salt and Pepper to taste

Method

Combine all ingredients in a bowl and mix it well.

Yield:

2 servings

Appetizers and Snacks

Here we have a pick of the best vegan snack recipes that can be serves for Sunday brunches and family get-togethers.

Tofu Steaks with Red Pepper - Walnut Sauce

This dish transforms tofu into a crunchy snack that can be served with home-made walnut sauce for a nutty flavor.

Ingredients

- 1 (14-ounce) package water-packed reduced-fat extra-firm tofu
- 3 tbsps. chopped walnuts, toasted
- 1/4 cup finely chopped fresh basil
- 1 tbsp. Dijon mustard
- 1/2 tsp. crushed red pepper
- 8 garlic cloves, minced
- 1/2 cup all-purpose flour
- 1/2 cup egg substitute
- 2 cups panko (Japanese breadcrumbs)
- 2 tbsps. olive oil
- 1 (12-ounce) bottle roasted red peppers, drained
- 2 tbsps. chopped fresh parsley
- 1 tbsp. chopped fresh thyme
- 2 tbsps. white wine vinegar
- 1/4 cup water
- 1/4 tsp. salt

Method

1. Cut tofu crosswise into 4 slices. Place it on several layers of paper towels and cover it with layers of paper towels.
2. Let it remain for half an hour. Press it occasionally to drain the water.
3. Mix basil, 1/4 cup water, parsley, thyme, vinegar, mustard, 1/2 tsp. salt, red pepper and garlic in a bowl.
4. Marinate the tofu slices with this mix and refrigerate for an hour.
5. Take 3 small bowls and place them side by side. In one add the flour, in the second add egg substitute and in third add panko.
6. Remove tofu from the marinade, reserving the remaining marinade.
7. Take each tofu slice and coat it in the flour, egg substitute and panko in that order.
8. When all the slices are thus coated, place a skillet on medium heat and brown the tofu slices on each side.
9. Remove from the heat and keep it warm.
10. Add the reserved marinade, walnuts and bell peppers to a blender and blend it until smooth.
11. Pour this mix into a pan and heat it for 2 minutes. Serve it with tofu.

Portobello Fritte

This dish combines the succulence of portobello mushrooms with a savory wine sauce. The vegan butter gives it a smooth consistency. This dish looks and tastes great.

Ingredients

- 4 portobello mushrooms, stems removed
- 1/2 cup dry red wine
- 1/4 cup vegetable stock
- 1 tsp. minced shallots
- 1 tbsp. olive oil
- 1 tsp. minced fresh garlic
- 1/2 tsp. salt, divided
- 1/2 tsp. black pepper, divided
- 1tsp. Dijon mustard
- 1 tsp. water
- 1 tbsp. vegan butter
- 1 tbsp. chopped tarragon
- 1/4 tsp. cornstarch
- 2 tbsps. canola oil
- 2 baked potatoes, cooled and cut lengthwise into 8 wedges each

Method

1. Pre heat oven to 400F.
2. Mix olive oil, garlic, shallots,1/4 tsp. salt and ¼ tsp. pepper in a bowl.
3. Add the mushrooms and coat it gently on all sides. Take a baking pan and arrange the mushrooms cap side down, at the bottom.
4. Bake it for about 12 minutes. Remove from the oven. Place 1 mushroom in each of 4 plates.
5. Add wine, vegetable stock and mustard to the baking pan.
6. Stir well to mix with the mushroom juices. Pour this mixture into a saucepan over medium heat.
7. Bring it to a boil and cook until the wine mixture is reduced to ¼ cup. Mix 1 tsp. water and corn-starch with a whisk.
8. Add the corn flour mixture to the wine mixture and boil until the mixture becomes thick.
9. Add vegan butter and tarragon and stir well.
10. Place a skillet over medium heat. Add the canola oil.
11. Add potato wedges and brown each side. Garnish with salt and pepper and serve with mushrooms and wine sauce.

Yield: 4 servings

South West Puff Pastry Bites

This snack is easy to make and tasty too.

Ingredients

- 1 tbsp. Olive Oil
- 3 tbsps. of Sweet Corn (canned)
- ¼ cup of Kidney Beans (canned)
- 1 medium White Onion (diced)
- ½ Green Bell Pepper (diced)
- 1 Garlic Clove (minced)
- ½ cup Water
- ½ Avocado (sliced)
- 1 tbsp. of Tomato Paste
- ¼ tsp. Cayenne Pepper
- ½ tsp. Salt
- ½ tsp. Cumin
- 1 tsp. Thyme
- 1 tsp. Paprika
- 1 sheet of Puff Pastry

Method

1. Pre heat oven to 400F and line the cookie sheet with baking paper.
2. Place a skillet on medium heat and add olive oil .Add bell pepper, onion and garlic and sauté until onions are soft.
3. Add the corn and beans and stir well. Add water and tomato paste. Mix well and season with the spices and herbs.
4. Simmer over low heat for 5 minutes.
5. Cut puff pastry sheet into 2 inch squares and arrange them on the baking paper.
6. Top each square with a tsp. of the mixture and bake for 15 minutes. Remove from the oven and serve with a slice of avocado on top.

Yield

4 Servings

Vegetable and Garlic Stuffed Mushrooms

This is a snack that is juicy and filled with flavor.

Ingredients

- 15 Mushrooms (Cremini) washed, stem removed and hollowed
- 1 tsp. of Olive Oil
- 1 Shallot ,diced
- 1 small bunch of Chives ,diced
- 1 Red Bell Pepper
- 3 Garlic cloves (crushed)
- ½ tsp. of Salt
- ¼ tsp. of Pepper
- Olive Oil
- Fresh Parsley leaves

Method

1. Pre heat oven to 480F.
2. Place the hollowed mushrooms in a baking dish.
3. Slice the parts of the mushroom that were removed and place it in a bowl.
4. Add shallot, chives, garlic, bell pepper, I tsp. olive oil, pepper and salt and mix well.
5. Spoon the mixture into the hollowed mushrooms to fill them. Sprinkle mushrooms with olive oil.
6. Cover the baking dish with a foil and bake for about 15-20 minutes. Garnish with parsley and serve.

Yield

15 stuffed mushrooms

Vegan Spinach Balls

Spinach is a power food that contains proteins, minerals, vitamins and iron. It is helps in skin, hair and bone health. Here is a snack that will make you relish your greens.

Ingredients

- 3 cups (3 ounces) Fresh Spinach (washed and dried)
- 1 Chia or Flax Egg
- 1 small Red Onion (quartered)
- ½ cup Cashews (whole and raw)
- 1 cup Almonds (whole and raw)
- 3 tbsps. Olive Oil
- ½ tsp. Salt
- ½ cup Oats

Method

1. Preheat oven to 350F and line cookie sheet with parchment paper.
2. Take a blender and add all the ingredients and blend it until the nuts are slightly ground.
3. Remove from the oven. Make tbsp. sized balls out of this spinach mixture.
4. Place it on the cookie sheet and bake for approximately 15-20 minutes, until the bottom turns brown.
5. Remove from the oven and serve warm.

Yield

20 servings

Beluga Black Lentil Burgers

Beluga lentils are rich in proteins and easy to prepare. They retain their shape after cooking. Sweet potatoes are rich in anti-oxidants, vitamins, minerals and dietary fiber. This is a healthy burger that you can make for your family.

Ingredients

- ½ cup uncooked Beluga Lentils
- 1 large Sweet Potato (steamed)
- 3 large Garlic cloves (crushed)
- 1 small Carrot (grated)
- ½ cup vegan Bread Crumbs
- ½ cup fresh Parsley (chopped)
- 1 tsp. Cumin
- Olive Oil
- ½ tsp. Salt
- ¼ tsp. Pepper

Method

Preheat oven to 440F.

Steam sweet potatoes until it becomes soft and keep it aside. Keep a stock pot on medium heat and add a cup of water to it. Add the lentils and bring to a boil. Let it simmer for half an hour.

Take a mixing bowl. Peel the sweet potato and mash it up. Add carrots, garlic and parsley and mix well. Add the cooked lentils and bread crumbs. Mix well. Make 12 patties of 3 to 4 inches.

Line a baking dish with parchment paper and arrange the patties at the bottom. Sprinkle olive oil and bake for 15 minutes. Flip the patties and bake the other side for another 10 minutes.

Remove the patties from oven and place it on burger bun and serve with tomatoes, onion and avocado.

Yield

12 Servings

Coconut Beet Patties

Beets contain antioxidants that help fight diseases. Coconuts contain iron, zinc, protein and fiber. This dish is a healthy combination of beets and coconuts and scores high on the taste quotient.

Ingredients

- 1 large Beet
- ¼ cup Shredded coconut
- ¼ cup vegan Bread Crumbs
- ¼ tsp. Garlic Powder
- ¼ cup Whole Wheat Flour
- 6 tbsps. Water
- 1 tbsp. Olive Oil
- Mango Vinaigrette
- ¼ tsp. Salt

Method

1. Peel and steam beet for 35-50 minutes until soft. Keep it aside.
2. Take a plate and mix bread crumbs, shredded coconut, salt and garlic powder.
3. In another plate, mix flour and water to form a thick paste. Slice the beets into ½ inch slices.
4. Take each beet slice and dip it first in the flour mixture and then the coconut-bread crumb mixture.
5. Make sure all the slices are well-coated.
6. Pour 1 tbsp. of olive oil into a skillet and place it over medium heat.
7. Fry the patties on each side until it turns golden brown. Serve with mango vinaigrette.

Yield

6 patties

Tempeh Stuffed Butternut Squash

Butternut squash is very high on the health quotient and fortifies the immune system. It can protect your body from illnesses. This dish can be a nutritious snack for your family.

Ingredients

- 8 ounces Tempeh (diced)
- 1 Butternut Squash (cut into half)
- 1 Bell Pepper (diced)
- 3 tbsps. Olive Oil
- ½ cup Tomato Puree
- 1 medium Tomato (diced)
- 1 medium Onion (diced)
- 2 cloves of Garlic (crushed)
- 1 tbsp. of Pure Maple Syrup
- ½ cup of fresh Parsley (chopped)
- Cayenne Pepper

Method

Heat oven to 395F.Halve the squash, remove the seeds and grease the cut side with olive oil. Line a baking dish with baking paper. Place the squash cut side down in the dish. Cook for 40-45 minutes until the squash becomes soft.

Place a skillet on medium heat and add olive oil. Sauté the tempe and onion till the onions become soft and the tempeh turns slightly brown. Add tomato, tomato puree, bell pepper and maple syrup. Add salt and cayenne pepper for seasoning. Reduce the heat and let it warm.

Remove the butternut squash from the oven and hollow it out leaving only the edges. Fill the tempeh mixture into the hollow of the squash, sprinkle olive oil and cook in the oven for about 10 minutes. Take the squash out of the oven, top it with parsley, cut into 3-4 pieces and serve as an appetizer.

Yield

5   servings

Sweet Potato Burgers

Sweet potatoes are readily available, inexpensive, delicious and nutritious. These burgers can be quickly put together as an evening snack. They are yummy when combined with yogurt sauce.

Ingredients

Burgers

- ½ a Sweet Potato (peeled, diced)
- 1 White Onion (chopped well)
- 2 tbsps. of Olive Oil
- 1 large clove of Garlic (crushed)
- ¼ tsp. of Cumin
- ½ tsp. of Salt
- 2 tbsps. of Sweet Corn
- ½ tsp. of Thyme
- 1 tsp. of Paprika
- 3 tbsps. of Kidney Beans (or other type of bean)
- 6 tbsps. Breadcrumbs
- 6 burger buns

"Yogurt" Sauce

- ¼ cup of Plain Soy Yogurt
- Black Pepper
- Oregano
- Cumin
- Cayenne Pepper
- Salt to taste

Method

Preheat oven to 435F.

Place a frying pan over medium heat and add the olive oil. Add onion, garlic and sweet potato and sauté for a few minutes. Cover and cook until the sweet potatoes turn soft. Scoop out the contents of the pan into a bowl. Add the spices and mix well and set it aside. When it has cooled, add beans, breadcrumbs and corn and mix well with your hands. Make 6 medium sized patties with the mix.

Take a baking pan, line it with parchment paper and place the patties on it. Bake it for about 15 minutes on each side.

Combine the yogurt with the spices to make the yogurt sauce. Remove the patties from the oven and place it on the bottom side of a burger bun. Add tomatoes, onions lettuce and yogurt sauce and cover with the top half. Repeat with the remaining 5 patties. The burgers are done.

Yield

6 Burgers

Vegan Egg Rolls

This is a snack with a Chinese flavor. Prepare in advance to make this dish, since it requires many ingredients. This would be an ideal snack during weekends.

Ingredients

- 1 cup chopped fresh wood ear or shiitake mushrooms
- 1 cup shredded carrots
- 1 tsp. kosher salt
- 1tbsp. pinkpeppercorns, crushed
- 1cup Chinese red rice vinegar
- 2 ounces bean threads
- 1/2 tbsps. toasted sesame oil
- 1 1/2 tsp. plus 1 tbsp. vegetable oil
- 1 1/2 qts. thinly sliced cabbage
- About 18 fresh egg roll wrappers (5 in. square)
- 1/2 tsp. pepper
- 3tbsps.sugar
- 1/3 cup ketchup

Method

1. Take a sauce pan and place it over low heat.
2. Add peppercorns, sugar and vinegar and simmer until the vinegar is reduced to half.
3. Add the ketchup and strain the mix and place it in the freezer.
4. Drop the noodles into very hot water, and let it remain for 4 minutes. Drain it, cut it up a little bit and set it aside.
5. Keep a frying pan over medium heat and add the sesame oil and 1 ½ tsp. vegetable oil. Add carrots, mushrooms, cabbage, salt and pepper and cook until the vegetables are wilted. Add the cooked noodles and mix well.
6. Pre heat oven to 450F.
7. Lay the egg roll wrapper on the kitchen table with a corner facing you.
8. Spoon in about a quarter cup of filling just below the center.
9. Lift the top and bottom corners over the filling and then fold in the sides to the top corner to seal it.
10. Repeat with the remaining egg rolls. When all the egg rolls are filled, arrange them on a baking dish over a parchment paper.
11. Brush the sides of the rolls with the 1 tbsp. vegetable oil.
12. Bake the rolls, turning occasionally, until browned. This may take about 20 minutes. Halve the rolls and serve with sauce.

Yield

18   spring rolls

Avocado Hummus

Avocado hummus with pita bread can be a good evening snack for your family. The hummus is savory and can be used as a spread on sandwiches.

Ingredients

- 1½ cups Chickpeas (rinsed and drained from a can or soaked and cooked)
- 1 Avocado
- small handful fresh Cilantro
- 2 tbsps. fresh Lime Juice
- 5 tbsps. Water
- ½ tsp. Salt
- 1 - 2 Garlic Cloves (optional)
- Red Pepper Flakes (optional)

Method

1. Pulse together all the ingredients in a blender.
2. Garnish with red pepper flakes and serve with vegetables or pita bread.

Quick Roasted Garlic bread

Make bread more interesting for your family by following this simple recipe.

Ingredients

- Crusty Bread – 1 loaf
- Salt
- Pepper
- Garlic powder
- Olive oil

Method

1. Pre heat your oven to 400F.Line a baking pan with baking paper.
2. Slice the bread into thin slices. You will get about 20 slices. Sprinkle salt, garlic powder and pepper and give it a touch of olive oil.
3. Flip the bread over to garnish the other side. Repeat for all the remaining slices.
4. Bake in the upper part of the oven for 10 minutes. Serve with soup.

Yield

20 slices of garlic bread

Desserts

You can impress your family and friends with some wonderful dessert recipes that are 100% vegan.

Banana-Oat Cups

Serves: 6 | Prep Time: ~ 35 min |

WHAT YOU NEED:

- 2 ½ cups old-fashioned rolled oats
- 3 cups water
- 1% cups almond milk (see recipe)
- ½ cup flaxseeds (ground)
- ½ cup chia seeds
- 2 bananas (medium, sliced)

- 2-5 tsp. cinnamon powder (to taste)
- 4 tsp. Himalayan salt (more or less to taste)
- 1 stick vanilla (crushed)

Total number of what you need: 10

HOW YOU MAKE IT:

1. Soak the chia seeds in a cup of water at room temperature.

2. Drain excess water after soaking the seeds for about 10-30 minutes.

3. Toast the rolled oats in a medium pot on medium heat.

4. Add the water, almond milk, flaxseeds and chia seeds to the toasted rolled oats.

5. Stir well and bring the mixture to a boil over medium low heat.

6. Once boiling, turn the stove down to low heat and, add in the bananas, cinnamon and a pinch of salt.

7. Stir the mixture well, while cooking slowly for about 10 minutes or until the desired consistency is reached.

8. Once the heat is turned off, add the vanilla extract and stir once more.

9. Take off the stove and let the mixture chill until cooled down.

10. Serve in a cup or pour into a mason jar for storage and enjoy!

Raspberry Lemon Ice-Cream

Serves: 5 | Prep Time: ~90 min |

WHAT YOU NEED:

- 1 cup water

- 1 tsp. psyllium husk

- 1 organic lemon with peel

- 1 can full-fat coconut milk

- Pinch of stevia

- 1 cup raspberries

Total number of what you need: 6

HOW YOU MAKE IT:

1. Combine 1 cup of water with the psyllium husk in small pan over medium heat.

2. Stir thoroughly until the psyllium husk and water form a gel-like consistency.

3. Take about 1 tablespoon of lemon zest from the fresh lemon.

4. Combine the coconut milk, stevia, raspberries, tablespoon of lemon zest and all the lemon juice of the lemon with the psyllium husk mixture in a blender.

5. Blend the ingredients for about 3 minutes, until desired consistency is reached.

6. Transfer the mixture to a bowl. Transfer this bowl to the fridge and chill it for 1 hour.

7. Pour the mix into an ice-cream maker. Alternatively, pour all but ½ cup of the blended mixture into an ice cube tray and freeze it. After this part of the mixture is frozen, blend the cubes of mixture with the ½ cup unfrozen mixture to create delicious ice-cream.

8. Enjoy right away and/or store the ice cream in a container!

Mexikale Crisps

Serves: 2 | Prep Time: ~10 min |

WHAT YOU NEED:

- 8 cups kale leaves (large, chopped)

- 1 tsp. garlic powder

- 1 tsp. ground cumin

- ½ tsp. chili powder

- 1 tsp. dried oregano

- 1 tsp. dried cilantro

- Himalayan salt and pepper to taste

Total number of what you need: 9

HOW YOU MAKE IT:

1. Preheat the oven to 350°F or 175°C.

2. Line a baking tray with parchment paper and set it aside.

3. Absorb any remaining water from the chopped kale leaves with paper towels.

4. Place the chopped leaves in a large bowl and add the seasonings.

5. Mix and shake well before adding more seasonings if desired. Mix all the ingredients again.

6. Spread out the kale chips on the baking tray.

7. Bake the kale in the oven for 10-15 minutes. Check every minute after the 10-minute mark until the preferred crispiness is reached.

8. Take the tray out of the oven and set it aside to cool down.

9. Serve and enjoy or store in a container for later!

Black Bean & Quinoa Burgers

Serves: 3 | Prep Time: ~40 min |

WHAT YOU NEED:

- 1 cup dry black beans

- ½ cup dry quinoa

- ½ purple onion (chopped)

- ¼ cup bell pepper (any color, seeded and chopped)

- 2 tablespoons garlic (minced)

- ½ cup whole wheat flour

- ½ tsp. red pepper flakes

- ½ tsp. paprika

- 1 tsp. Himalayan salt

- 1 tsp. pepper

- 4-6 large leaves of lettuce

- Roasted sesame seeds (optional)

Total number of what you need: 13

HOW YOU MAKE IT:

1.   Prepare the beans according to the method.

2.   Prepare the quinoa according to the recipe.

3.   Preheat the oven to 350°F or 175°C.

4.   Put a non-stick frying pan over medium-high heat, and then add the onions, bell peppers, garlic, salt, and pepper.

5.   Stir-fry until the ingredients begin to soften, for about 5 minutes. Remove the pan from the heat and let it cool down for about 10 minutes.

6.   Once the veggies have cooled down, put them in a food processor along with the cooked beans, quinoa, flour, and remaining spices; pulse until it's a chunky mixture.

7.   Lay out a baking pan covered with parchment paper and form the blended mixture into 6 evenly-sized patties.

8.   Place the patties on the pan and place them in the freezer for about 5 minutes to prevent crumbling.

9.   Take out the pan from the fridge and put it in the oven until the patties have browned, in about 15 minutes.

10.   Serve each burger wrapped in a lettuce leaf (or burger bun) and, if desired, top with the optional roasted sesame seeds. Alternatively, store to enjoy later.

Peanut Butter Brownies

Serves: 8 | Prep Time: ~15 min |

WHAT YOU NEED:

- 1 ½ cups water (lukewarm)

- 1/2 cup organic peanut butter (see recipe)

- ½ cup cocoa powder

- 2 tsp. baking powder

- 2 scoops pea protein powder

- 2 tbsp. coconut flour

- ½ cup almonds (optional)

Total number of what you need: 7

HOW YOU MAKE IT:

1. Preheat the oven to 350°F or 175°C.

2. Take a medium bowl and mix the lukewarm water and peanut butter into a smooth mixture.

3. Take another medium bowl and mix the cocoa powder, baking powder, vegan protein powder and coconut flour. Mix the ingredients well to avoid any remaining lumps.

4. Add the first mixture to the second mixture and combine both into a batter.

5. Pour the batter into a slightly greased oven dish, optionally lined with parchment paper.

6. Let the mixture bake for 40-45 minutes, until a knife comes out of the center clean.

7. Take out the oven dish and allow the brownie chunk to cool down before cutting it into 8 brownies.

8. Enjoy, share or store!

Vegan Blueberry Lime Cheese Cake

This is a dish that will be relished by your family. It contains the goodness of berries that have powerful antioxidant properties.

Ingredients

- 1 cup fresh Blueberries
- 4 Medjool Dates
- 2 cups Coconut Cream
- ⅔ cups Cashews (soaked in water for 10-15 minutes)
- 1 cup Macadamia Nuts (raw, unsalted)
- 4tbsps.Fresh Lime Juice
- 2 tbsps. Maple Syrup
- 2 Medjool Dates
- 1 tsp. Lime Zest
- ½ cup fresh Blueberries
- Pinch of Salt

Method

1. Take a 7-inch spring form and line it with parchment paper.
2. Mix Macadamia nuts, 4 Mejdool dates and a pinch of salt in a blender and blend until you get a thick, sticky mix.
3. Press the mix inside the spring form to form the crust and work it halfway up the sides with your finger.
4. Place this crust in the freezer while you get to work on the filling.
5. In the blender, mix maple syrup, coconut cream, cashews and lime juice and blend it well.
6. Remove the spring form from the refrigerator and pour the filling inside it.
7. Once again, place the spring form in the freezer until the filling is slightly firm. This may take 10 minutes.
8. Clean out the blender and add 1 cup blueberries and 2 dates and blend well. Spread the blueberry topping on top of the filling.

9. Refrigerate for a minimum of 4 hours. Garnish with fresh blue berries and lime zest and serve.

Yield

8 servings

Vegan Chocolate Strawberry Cupcakes

Chocolates are an all-time favorite with adults and children alike. Here is a winning combination of chocolate and strawberry to titillate your taste buds.

Ingredients

- 1/2 cups flour
- 1/3 cup unsweetened cocoa powder
- 1/2 tsp. salt
- 1/2 cup vegetable oil
- 1 cup sugar
- 1 tsp. baking soda
- 2 tbsps. distilled white vinegar
- 2 tsp. vanilla extract

Frosting and Finishing

- 1 1/2 cups sliced strawberries
- About 4 tbsp. nondairy milk, such as soy, almond, or rice
- 2 tsp. vanilla extract
- 2/3 cup nonhydrogenated vegetable shortening
- 2 2/3 cups plus 1 tbsp. sifted powdered sugar

Method

Preheat oven to 350F. Take a 12-cup muffin pan and line it with cupcake liners.

Take a bowl and mix the flour, cocoa, sugar, salt and baking soda and whisk well. In another bowl whip up the vinegar, oil and vanilla. Combine the two mixtures in a larger bowl and mix well. Fill the batter into the cupcake cups and bake for 15-10 minutes. Allow the cupcakes to cool.

Frosting: Add 2 2/3 cup powdered sugar and vanilla extract to your blender and blend on high for a few minutes. Whisk in the non-dairy milk 1 tsp. at a time and keep whisking it to get a smooth, fluffy mixture.

Cut the tops off the cupcakes and keep it aside. Place 1 tbsp. of frosting on top of each cupcake and smooth it out. Cover with a few strawberries and replace the top. Strain the remaining 1 tbsp. powdered sugar using a fine-mesh strainer and sprinkle on top of the cupcake.

Yield

12 cupcakes

Vegan Mint Chocolate Mousse

This delectable dish combines the richness of chocolate with the freshness and flavor of mint.

Ingredients

- 6 tbsps. Cacao or unsweetened cocoa
- 1½ cups Coconut Milk
- Vegan Chocolate Chips
- ¼ tsp. Peppermint Extract

Method
1. Whisk together the cacao, coconut milk and mint extract until bubbles appear.
2. Pour into 2 ramekins and keep in the refrigerator for a minimum of 4 hours.
3. Remove from the refrigerator when the mousse is set. Sprinkle chocolate chips on top and serve.

Yield
2 servings

Vegan Peanut Butter Mousse Pie

Here is a dessert that is tasty and gives you the proteins that your body needs.

Ingredients

- 1 cup Natural Peanut Butter

- 2 cups Walnuts halves
- 2 tbsps. unsweetened Cocoa Powder
- 18 Dates or 10 Medjool Dates
- 2 cups Coconut Cream (chilled)
- 2 tbsps. Maple Syrup
- ¼ cup Vegan Chocolate Chips (melted)
- A pinch of Salt

Method

1. Line a 7 inch pie form with parchment paper.
2. Mix the walnuts, dates, cocoa powder and salt in a blender and pulse it till you get a sticky mass.
3. Keep this at the bottom of the pie form and press it firmly in place.
4. Place it in the freezer to form the pie crust.
5. Blend the coconut cream, peanut butter and maple syrup in the blender until you get a creamy, soft mixture.
6. Remove the pie crust from the freezer and spread the peanut butter mousse on the crust.
7. Melt chocolate chips in a microwave and top it over the mousse.

Yield

1 pie

Apple Banana Muffins (with Streusel)

Here is a fruity dessert that your family will love. It combines the apple with the tropical banana to give a dessert that is as nutritious as it is tasty.

Ingredients

- 1 Apple (peeled, pitted, and diced)
- 2 Bananas (pureed)
- ½ cup of Walnut Halves (chopped)
- ½ cup of All Purpose Flour
- 1½ cup of Whole Wheat Flour
- 2 tbsps. of Raw Cane Sugar
- ½ cup of Walnut Halves (chopped)
- ½ cup of All Purpose Flour
- ¼ cup of Walnut Halves
- ⅓ cup of Rolled Oats
- 3 tbsps. of Coconut Oil
- ⅓ cup of Olive Oil
- ¾ cup Plant Based Milk
- ⅓ cup Raw Cane Sugar
- ½ tsp. of Baking Soda
- 1 tsp. of Baking Powder
- ¼ tsp. Salt
- ¼ tsp. of Cinnamon
- A pinch of Nutmeg

Method

1. Preheat oven to 350F.Line a muffin tray with muffin cups.
2. Mix the milk, bananas and olive oil in a blender and blend to get a smooth mixture.
3. In a large bowl, mix the flours, baking soda, baking powder, 1/3 cup sugar, cinnamon, salt and nutmeg.
4. Add the blended banana/milk mixture to the bowl and combine well. Add the diced apple and chopped walnuts and mix once again.
5. Fill the muffin dough in the muffin cups.
6. Add walnuts, oats, coconut oil and 2 tbsps. sugar to the blender and pulse until mixed well.
7. Top the muffins with the streusel topping. Bake in your oven for 15-18 minutes. Allow it to cool and serve.

Yield

12 Servings

Vegan Coconut Banana Cheesecake

Here is a coconut delight that also has the sweetness of banana and the richness of peanuts.

Ingredients

- 1 Banana
- 1 cup Coconut Cream
- 1 cup Peanuts (roasted, lightly salted)
- 1½ tsp. Coconut Oil
- 1 tbsp. Pure Maple Syrup
- ⅓ cup Vegan Mini Chocolate Chips

Method

1. Line a 7 inch spring form with parchment paper. Pulse peanuts with coconut oil in a blender to form a crumbly mass.
2. Place this mix at the bottom of the spring form and press it down firmly to form the crust.
3. Clean the blender and pulse banana, maple syrup and coconut cream to form a smooth mixture.
4. Spread this mixture over the peanut crust. Sprinkle coconut chips on top and place in the freezer for 10 minutes until it becomes firm.
5. Remove the cheesecake from the spring form and serve.

Yield

8   cheesecakes

Vegan Kiwi Mango Cheesecake

This is a tropical delight that combines two powerful fruits, mangoes and the kiwi fruit.

Ingredients

- 3 Kiwis (skin removed)
- ¾ cup Mangos (diced)
- 5 Medjool Dates
- ⅔ cup of Almonds (raw)
- 1 cup Coconut Cream
- ½ cup Cashew
- 2 tbsp. Powdered Sugar
- 2 Medjool Dates
- A pinch of Salt
- 1 tbsp. Lime Juice

Method

1. Line a 7 inch spring form with parchment paper.
2. Add almonds, 5 dates and salt to your blender and pulse to form a sticky mass.
3. Place this mix at the bottom of the spring form and press down to form the crust.
4. Place it in the freezer and allow it to get set.
5. Rinse the blender and add the cashews, kiwi, coconut cream, powdered sugar and lime juice.
6. Pulse until you get a smooth mixture. Remove the spring form from the freezer and fill the crust with this kiwi-cheesecake mix.
7. Rinse the blender again and add the mango and 2 dates and pulse to form a smooth mix.
8. Top the filling with this mix. Refrigerate for a minimum of 4 hours.
9. When the cheesecake is ready, remove from the refrigerator, garnish with mint leaves and kiwi slices and serve.

Yield:

8 servings

Nut Butter Cranberry Cookies

Nut butter and cranberries make an interesting combination and these delicious, crunchy cookies can make a wonderful dessert or snack dish.

Ingredients

- ½ cup of Nut Butter (Almond Butter or Peanut Butter)
- ⅔ cup Dried Cranberries (chopped)
- ½ cup of Raw Cane Sugar
- 1 cup of Whole Wheat Flour
- 1 Chia Egg
- 2 tbsps. of Coconut Oil

Method

1. Pre-heat oven to 300F.Take a bowl and add nut butter, coconut oil, sugar and chia egg.
2. Whisk it well to form a consistent mixture. Add the cranberries and whole wheat flour and mix well.
3. Roll the dough on a counter top to form a log of 5 inch length and 2 inch diameter.
4. Wrap this in a plastic wrap and place in the refrigerator for 45 minutes.
5. Remove the cookie log from the refrigerator and cut it into 10 cookie slices.
6. Arrange the cookies on a baking sheet and bake for about 20 minutes until the edges become golden brown. Allow it to cool and store in a container.

Yield

10 cookies

Conclusion

Going Plant Base in today's world can be tough. Restaurants don't have a Plant Based option and airlines don't offer these foods preferences. This is because nobody understands what it means to be a on a plant based diet, and sometimes even mistake it for vegetarianism. The common task of buying groceries can be excruciating because of the limited choices you have. Food should be easy; ordering Chinese takeout or going to a restaurant should not have to be the ordeal it is for your family.

In such a scenario, it is better to take matters into your own hands and cook—at least, until restaurant chains become open to including vegan options in their menus. The intent behind compiling these recipes was to give you a single space from which you can gain inspiration to cook that sumptuous plant based meal. These easy (and other not so easy) recipes can help you cook a full course meal for your family.

It doesn't matter what your family desires—some soup to combat a fever, a salad during a breezy get-together, desserts or even appetizers—this book has it all! The recipes were taken from multiple countries, in the hope that you get a taste of flavors from around the world. Why limit yourself to just what you know? Some recipes were included just for the kids, so they won't groan when you call them for dinner.

Now, meal time won't be about struggles at the grocer's and battling with bland tastes. No more making do with food that is not worthy of you or your family. No more elaborate experimentation with recipes that may or may not work for you.

Care was taken to ensure that the ingredients are easy to obtain and procure and follow through with the greenprint; most of the ingredients will be readily available in the local grocery store or nearest supermarket. Many of the recipes can be whipped up swiftly in a schedule that includes dropping the kids off at school and getting them from soccer practice. Others can be used for family dinners over the weekend. You can even cook a romantic, vegan meal for two when the kids have gone to your mother's.

It takes a lot of resolution and determination to undergo this greenprint diet, living this lifestyle and staying that way; kudos to you and your family for choosing the Plant based life and staying there, against all odds. I hope you find the recipes in this book useful. Happy Plant Base days ahead!

Thank You

If you follow religiously to <u>The Greenprint: Plant-Based Diet, Best Body, Better World By Marco Borges</u>. And some of the clean, and delicious plant based recipes provided for you in this book. You are going to be seeing great results in your body and health, because you will lose weight and keep it Off for good.

<u>If you enjoyed the recipes in this book, please take the time to share your thoughts and post a positive review with 5 star rating on Amazon, it would encourage me and make me serve you better. It'd be greatly appreciated!</u>

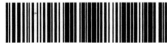

Made in the USA
Lexington, KY
25 January 2019